Coconut oil benefits

Different listed ways coconut oil help in keeping the hair and skin healthy

Dr walt wade

Contents

chapter1

introduction to coconut oil

Coconut oil has been gaining a lot of attention and popularity in recent years, with many health and wellness experts hailing it as a superfood with numerous benefits. It is extracted from the meat of mature coconuts and has been a staple in tropical regions for centuries. However, it has only been in the last decade or so that the western world has come to realize the many uses and benefits of this versatile oil. In this article, we will delve into the history, uses, and potential health benefits of coconut oil, as well as its nutritional value and different types available in the market. History of Coconut Oil Coconut oil has a long history of traditional use in various cultures, particularly in tropical regions such as Asia, Africa, and the Caribbean. The coconut palm tree, known scientifically as Cocos nucifera, is known as the "tree of life" as almost every part of the tree – from its fruit to its leaves – is utilized in some way. It is believed that the coconut palm originated in the Indian-Indonesian region and then spread to other tropical regions by the Indian Ocean. The earliest written records of the coconut tree can be traced back to the Hindu epic Ramayana, which dates back to 1500 BC. In traditional Ayurvedic medicine, coconut oil was used as a natural remedy for a wide range of health conditions, including skin and hair problems, as well as digestive issues. It was also used in cooking, as a natural moisturizer and sun protector for the skin, and even as a natural toothpaste. Uses of Coconut Oil Coconut oil is a highly versatile oil and has a wide range of practical, culinary, and cosmetic uses. In cooking, coconut oil is a popular and healthier alternative to traditional vegetable oils. It has a high smoke point, which means it can be used in high-heat cooking methods without losing its beneficial properties. It is also a plant-based source of saturated fats, which has been proven to have numerous health benefits. Besides cooking, coconut oil is also used in baking, as a substitute for butter or other cooking oils. Its neutral taste and creamy texture make it a perfect addition to baked goods, providing a unique, subtle coconut flavor. In the cosmetic industry, coconut oil is a common ingredient in skincare and hair care products. Its moisturizing properties make it an excellent natural skin and hair conditioner, and its antibacterial and anti-inflammatory properties make it effective in treating skin conditions such as eczema, psoriasis, and acne. Furthermore, coconut oil is used in traditional medicine to improve digestive health, boost metabolism and energy, and promote weight loss. It is also used in Ayurvedic medicine as a natural oil pulling agent for oral health. Potential Health Benefits of Coconut Oil The health benefits of coconut oil have been heavily studied in recent years, and the results have been quite promising. However, it is essential to note that most of these studies have been done on the medium-chain fatty acids found in coconut oil, particularly lauric acid, caprylic acid, and capric acid. One of the most significant benefits of coconut oil is its impact on heart health. Contrary to popular belief, coconut oil has been found to increase HDL (good) cholesterol levels and improve the ratio of HDL to LDL (bad) cholesterol. This can reduce the risk of heart disease and stroke. Moreover, coconut oil has been found to boost metabolism and promote weight loss. This can be attributed to its medium-chain fatty acids, which are known to be quickly metabolized by the liver, providing a quick source of energy and promoting fat burning. In addition, research has shown that coconut oil may have anti-inflammatory, antibacterial, and antifungal properties, making it effective in treating skin conditions, infections, and even gastrointestinal issues. Nutritional Value of Coconut Oil Coconut oil is a rich source of healthy fats, including medium-chain triglycerides (MCTs) and lauric acid. These fats are easily digested and have been linked to various health benefits, as mentioned earlier. It also contains vitamin E and traces of vitamin K and iron. One tablespoon (15 ml) of coconut oil provides 121 calories, 14 grams of fat, and no significant amounts of carbohydrates or protein. Although it is relatively high in calories and fat, when consumed in moderation, coconut oil can be a part of a healthy and balanced diet. Types of Coconut Oil There are several types of coconut oil available in the market, and it is essential to know the differences between them. Refined coconut oil is produced by drying the coconut meat or copra, and then expeller-pressing, cooking, or applying solvents to extract the oil. This process removes the strong coconut aroma and flavor, making it a more neutral-tasting oil. However, this process also strips away some of the beneficial properties of the oil. On the other hand, virgin or unrefined coconut oil is extracted from fresh coconut meat without any high heat or chemical treatment. This type retains the strong aroma and flavor of coconut, as well as its nutritional value and beneficial properties. Another type of coconut oil is called fractionated coconut oil, which is extracted only from the medium-chain fatty acids of coconut oil. This results in an odorless, colorless liquid that remains liquid at room temperature, making it easier to use for culinary and cosmetic purposes. Conclusion In conclusion, coconut oil is a versatile oil with a long history of traditional use and potentially numerous health benefits. It is commonly used for cooking and baking, as well as in skincare and hair care products. Its unique nutritional profile and compatibility with various diets make it a popular choice among health enthusiasts. However, it is essential to note that coconut oil should be incorporated into a healthy and balanced diet, along with regular exercise and proper medical care, to reap its benefits fully. With its various uses and potential health benefits, coconut oil is undoubtedly a valuable addition to anyone's pantry or beauty routine.

chapter2

coconut oil for skin

Extracted from the meat of mature coconuts, coconut oil contains a unique combination of fatty acids that have anti-inflammatory and antibacterial properties. These properties make it an excellent solution for a range of skin conditions and concerns. Its rich texture and versatility make it a cost-effective and natural alternative to traditional skin care products. In this article, we will explore the numerous benefits that coconut oil provides when used on the skin. First and foremost, coconut oil is an excellent moisturizer. It has a high concentration of fatty acids, including lauric acid, which penetrates deep into the skin, making it soft and supple. It creates a protective layer over the skin that helps to retain moisture, preventing the skin from becoming dry and flaky. This makes it particularly beneficial for individuals with dry skin or those living in cold or dry climates. Coconut oil is also beneficial for those with oily or acne-prone skin. Many people believe that applying oil to the face can cause breakouts, but with coconut oil, that is not the case. It helps regulate the production of sebum, the skin's natural oil, and reduces the appearance of oily skin. Its antibacterial properties can also fight against acne-causing bacteria, helping to clear up pimples and prevent new ones from forming. Another benefit of coconut oil for skin is its anti-aging properties. It contains antioxidants that can help combat the damaging free radicals that cause early signs of aging such as wrinkles and fine lines. When applied topically, coconut oil can help reduce the appearance of these signs of aging by promoting collagen production and improving skin elasticity. Aside from its moisturizing and anti-aging benefits, coconut oil has a wide range of uses for treating specific skin conditions. For example, it can soothe eczema and psoriasis symptoms due to its anti-inflammatory properties. Its antibacterial and anti-fungal properties also make it an effective treatment for fungal infections and reduce redness and irritation caused by skin conditions such as rosacea. Coconut oil is also an excellent option for those with sensitive skin. It is gentle and non-irritating, making it suitable for all skin types, including those with sensitive skin. It can be used to soothe and calm skin that has been irritated by harsh chemicals or environmental factors. One of the most convenient aspects of using coconut oil for skin care is its versatility. Users can mix it with other natural ingredients, such as essential oils and honey, to create a personalized and effective skin care routine. For example, mixing coconut oil with honey can create a hydrating face mask, while adding a few drops of lavender essential oil can create a calming moisturizer. Coconut oil can also act as a natural makeup remover. It can effectively remove makeup, including waterproof products, without drying out the skin. Simply apply a small amount of coconut oil to a cotton pad and gently wipe away your makeup. This eliminates the need for harsh makeup removers that can strip the skin of its natural oils. In addition to its benefits for the skin, coconut oil has a pleasant scent that can uplift and relax the mind. It is often used in aromatherapy and has been proven to have a positive impact on mental health and well-being. Applying coconut oil to the skin can provide a calming and soothing experience, making it an excellent addition to self-care routines. When purchasing coconut oil for skin care, it's essential to opt for organic, unrefined, and cold-pressed varieties. This ensures that the oil has not gone through any chemical processes, preserving its natural properties. Additionally, it's best to store coconut oil in a cool and dry place to prevent it from melting and losing its beneficial properties.

chapter3

coconut oil for hair

One of the most significant benefits of coconut oil for hair is its ability to deeply moisturize and nourish the hair. Unlike many store-bought hair products that contain harmful chemicals, coconut oil is an all-natural solution that contains fatty acids that penetrate the hair shaft and provide hydration and nourishment from within. This makes it an excellent treatment for dry and damaged hair, as it helps restore and maintain the hair's natural moisture balance. In addition to its moisturizing properties, coconut oil also has antibacterial and antifungal properties, making it effective in treating and preventing scalp infections. A healthy scalp is crucial for beautiful and healthy hair growth, and coconut oil can help keep the scalp clean and free from bacterial and fungal infections that can lead to hair problems such as dandruff and hair loss. Coconut oil is also rich in lauric acid, a type of fatty acid that has been shown to have a significant impact on hair health. When applied to the hair, lauric acid binds to the hair proteins, strengthening the hair shaft and preventing breakage. This makes coconut oil an excellent choice for those with weak and brittle hair or anyone looking to grow their hair longer. But the benefits of coconut oil for hair go beyond just external application. Consuming coconut oil has been linked to improving overall hair health as well. The healthy fats and antioxidants found in coconut oil can help support hair growth, prevent hair loss, and even improve the appearance and shine of the hair. Adding a tablespoon of coconut oil to your diet can provide your hair with the essential nutrients it needs to thrive. Coconut oil can also protect the hair from damage caused by environmental factors such as sun exposure and pollution. The fatty acids in coconut oil form a protective layer around the hair, shielding it from the harmful UV rays of the sun and other damaging elements. This is especially important for those with color-treated or chemically processed hair, as coconut oil can help maintain the hair's color and prevent it from becoming dull and brittle. For those struggling with frizzy and unmanageable hair, coconut oil can be a game-changer. The fatty acids in coconut oil help to smooth the hair cuticle, reducing frizz and leaving the hair feeling soft and smooth. This makes it an excellent option for those with curly and coarse hair, as it can help define and enhance natural curls while keeping frizz at bay. Incorporating coconut oil into your hair care routine is also a cost-effective option. Many store-bought hair products can be expensive and contain harmful chemicals that can damage the hair over time. Coconut oil, on the other hand, is affordable and widely available, making it a budget-friendly alternative for those looking to improve their hair health. When using coconut oil for hair, it is essential to choose a high-quality, organic product. This ensures that you are getting all the natural benefits of coconut oil without any additives or chemicals. To use coconut oil as a hair treatment, warm a small amount in your palms and apply it to damp or dry hair, focusing on the ends. You can also use it as a pre-shampoo treatment by applying it to your hair and leaving it on for 30 minutes before washing it out. Coconut oil can also be used as a leave-in conditioner. By applying a small amount to the ends of your hair, you can add moisture and hydration without leaving your hair feeling greasy or weighed down. This is especially beneficial for those with dry and damaged hair, as it provides long-lasting moisture and nourishment throughout the day.

 coconut oil capsules

What are Coconut Oil Capsules? Coconut oil capsules are dietary supplements that contain a concentrated form of coconut oil. They are made by encapsulating coconut oil in a gelatin or vegetarian-based shell, making it easy to swallow and digest. These capsules are a popular alternative to traditional liquid coconut oil, which can sometimes have a strong flavor and odor that can be off-putting to some individuals. The coconut oil used in capsules is typically extracted from the meat of mature coconuts, which is then refined, filtered and encapsulated to create a concentrated form of the oil. Some manufacturers may also use cold-pressed or virgin coconut oil, which is considered to be of higher quality and contains more nutrients. Health Benefits of Coconut Oil Capsules Coconut oil has been praised for its many health benefits, and the same applies to its capsule form. Here are some of the significant advantages of consuming coconut oil capsules: 1. Boosts Cardiovascular Health: Coconut oil contains healthy fats that are known to increase the levels of HDL or good cholesterol in the body. At the same time, it also helps reduce the levels of LDL or bad cholesterol, thus promoting a healthy balance and reducing the risk of cardiovascular diseases. 2. Aids in Weight Loss: Coconut oil capsules are often marketed as a supplement for weight loss due to its medium-chain triglycerides (MCTs) content. MCTs are easily digested, provide longer satiety, and are not stored as fat in the body, making it an excellent alternative to traditional cooking oils. 3. Improves Brain Function: The MCTs in coconut oil are also believed to have beneficial effects on brain health. They can quickly enter the brain and provide a source of energy for the brain cells, thus improving cognitive function. 4. Fights Inflammation and Oxidative Stress: Coconut oil is rich in antioxidants, which help fight inflammation and oxidative stress in the body. Regular consumption of coconut oil capsules may help reduce the risk of chronic diseases like heart disease, cancer, and Alzheimer's. 5. Promotes Healthy Skin and Hair: Coconut oil has been used for centuries as a natural beauty treatment. It is rich in lauric acid, a fatty acid with excellent moisturizing properties that can improve skin and hair health. Consuming coconut oil capsules may promote a healthy scalp, reduce dandruff, and improve hair growth. 6. Aids in Managing Diabetes: Studies have shown that the MCTs in coconut oil can improve insulin sensitivity and reduce blood sugar levels. This makes coconut oil capsules a beneficial supplement for individuals with diabetes. How to Use Coconut Oil Capsules Coconut oil capsules are easy to use, and there are no strict guidelines for their consumption. The recommended dosage may vary from brand to brand, but it is generally recommended to take 1-2 capsules daily with a meal. It is essential to follow the instructions on the packaging and consult with a healthcare provider before starting any new supplement. Possible Side Effects of Coconut Oil Capsules Coconut oil capsules are generally considered safe for consumption, and they have very few side effects. Some individuals may experience minor side effects like upset stomach, diarrhea, or nausea when consuming coconut oil for the first time. This is usually due to the high fat content and can be avoided by starting with a smaller dosage and gradually increasing it. Coconut oil capsules are not recommended for individuals with allergies to coconut or those on blood-thinning medications. It is always advisable to consult with a healthcare provider before adding any new supplement to one's routine. Choosing the Right Coconut Oil Capsules When selecting coconut oil capsules, it is essential to look for a reputable brand that uses high-quality ingredients. The label should state the source of the coconut oil, and ideally, it should be organic, unrefined, and non-GMO. It is also important to check the amount of MCTs present in the capsules, as this directly affects their potency and benefits.

Coconut oil capsules offer a convenient and easy way to consume all the fantastic benefits of coconut oil. From promoting heart health and weight loss to improving skin and hair, these capsules have a range of potential benefits. When used in moderation and consumed as part of a well-balanced diet, coconut oil capsules can be a valuable addition to one's health and wellness routine. As with any supplement, it is advisable to consult with a healthcare provider before starting its use.

chapter4

coconut oil benefits

1. Boosts Immunity Coconut oil contains lauric acid, a medium-chain fatty acid that has anti-viral, anti-bacterial, and anti-fungal properties. When consumed, lauric acid is converted into monolaurin, a compound that helps to strengthen the immune system and fight off infections and diseases. Adding coconut oil to your diet can help you ward off illnesses and boost your immunity. 2. Promotes Heart Health Contrary to popular belief, saturated fats present in coconut oil are not harmful to our health. In fact, these fats can help to promote heart health by raising the levels of good cholesterol (HDL) in the body. This, in turn, can reduce the risk of heart disease and

stroke. Additionally, the antioxidants present in coconut oil also provide protection against heart damage caused by free radicals. 3. Aids in Weight Loss Coconut oil is a popular choice for those attempting to shed some pounds. This is because the medium-chain triglycerides (MCTs) present in coconut oil are metabolized differently in the body compared to other fats. These MCTs are quickly converted into energy instead of being stored in the body as fat. Additionally, coconut oil can help to reduce hunger and control cravings, making it an effective tool for weight loss. 4. Promotes Healthy Skin and Hair Coconut oil is a staple ingredient in many skin and haircare products, and for good reason. This oil is rich in fatty acids that provide deep moisturization to the skin and hair, making them soft, smooth, and hydrated. Its anti-inflammatory and antioxidant properties can also help to reduce redness, inflammation, and signs of aging. When used as a hair mask or leave-in conditioner, coconut oil can help to repair damaged hair and promote healthy hair growth. 5. Reduces Inflammation Inflammation is a natural response of the body to injury or infection, but chronic inflammation can lead to various health issues. Coconut oil contains compounds such as gallic acid and capric acid, which have anti-inflammatory properties. Regular consumption of coconut oil can help to reduce inflammation in the body and may also provide relief from conditions like arthritis. 6. Improves Brain Function Our brain requires a constant supply of energy in the form of glucose to function properly. However, as we age, our brain's ability to utilize glucose decreases, leading to cognitive decline and increased risk of neurodegenerative diseases like Alzheimer's. Coconut oil contains MCTs that can be easily converted into ketones, an alternative source of energy for the brain. This can help to improve brain function, memory, and focus, especially in older adults. 7. Helps to Control Blood Sugar Coconut oil may also be beneficial for those with diabetes or insulin resistance. MCTs present in coconut oil can improve insulin sensitivity and glucose tolerance, potentially helping to regulate blood sugar levels. Furthermore, studies have shown that consuming coconut oil can also increase the production of enzymes that aid in the breakdown of fats, which can be beneficial for those with diabetes or pre-diabetes. 8. Fights against Candida Infections Candida is a type of yeast that can cause infections in different parts of the body, such as the mouth, throat, and vagina. The medium-chain fatty acids in coconut oil, particularly caprylic acid, can help to combat candida overgrowth by disrupting the cell membranes of the yeast. This can help to eliminate the infection and prevent it from recurring. 9. Supports Digestive Health Coconut oil has a high content of medium-chain fatty acids, which are easier to digest compared to long-chain fatty acids. This makes it a great choice for those with digestive issues. Additionally, the anti-inflammatory and anti-microbial properties of coconut oil can also help to ease symptoms of conditions like irritable bowel syndrome (IBS) and improve gut health. 10. Natural Energy Booster Instead of reaching for a sugar-loaded energy drink, try incorporating coconut oil into your daily routine for a natural energy boost. As mentioned earlier, MCTs in coconut oil are quickly converted into energy by the body, providing a quick and sustained boost of energy. Adding a spoonful of coconut oil to your morning smoothie or coffee can help you start your day with a healthy and natural energy kick.

The end